©2018 - Penny Freeman Only For A Season - All Rights Reserved

Only For A Season

By Penny Freeman

Everyone has a story to tell, that one moment in time that can make or break you. This is the story of how you get through a tough season in life! It will offer guidance on what to do now that you have survived a catastrophic illness!

THIS BOOK IS DEDICATED TO MY SON, XIOME. WHO NEVER LETS ME DOWN, NEVER SEES MY FLAWS, AND ALWAYS ASSURES ME I WILL BE ALRIGHT, AS LONG AS, HE HAS BREATH! I LOVE YOU MORE THAN YOU WILL EVER KNOW!

MOM

TO MY SUPPORT TEAM, MY MOM AND DAD, MY AMAZING SISTERS, MY GRANDKIDS, AND MY FRIENDS...WORDS CANNOT EXPRESS THE LOVE AND JOY I HAVE RECEIVED FROM EACH OF YOU! I THANK YOU FROM THE BOTTOM OF MY HEART FOR HELPING ME IN THIS JOURNEY.

PENNY

CHAPTER 1

INTRODUCTION

On October 28, 2008, I suffered a ruptured brain aneurysm, there I said it! Funny how speaking it out loud seems to bring a sigh of relief or shock...still trying to figure that one out. It was alarming considering I was not sick, or on any medications. It came out of nowhere, and kicked my feet from under me! There were some warning signs but honestly, I thought it was just stress. BIG MISTAKE!

I remember believing that I could do anything, without consequences. You know things like, missing sleep, food binges, or just playing too hard! You would think that type of blind faith would serve a person well, but no, it is not always the case, so I found out! Instead, what I quickly realized was that life comes in seasons. Events that you must navigate, if you're going to succeed. Every season is a time of change, a time of alteration that requires you to do something! Your choices are given by what you decide is the best course of action with the circumstances life has given you. With that being said, I found a way of identifying the season I was in and how I could get through it. If I share my seasons, and what I did to prepare and often limit the difficulties as much as possible, then I have accomplished my goal...to help someone else navigate their seasons. I want to help you know that it is *only for a season* and you can get through it, with a little help.

To understand how I got here, I have to take you back to the beginning. No, not the moment I hit the earth, although that was filled with drama. But the beginning where I started to experience issues that could have played a part in the outcome of my life thus far. A memory that has stayed with me for so long. It is one of the few memories I still have. I believe it was a life-changing moment, one that started this roller-coaster ride, I was plunged into.

THE MEMORIES

In 1992, my ex-husband's father had died. I learned of this information from a friend who informed me that he was in town for the funeral. Since we had been divorced some 6 years, and we shared a son together, I had a sadness for him, since I knew his father.

We, were always, in a battle over how much time he spent with his son, or his lack of child support, since he did not live in town. To add insult to injury, he was constantly threatening to take my son away and I would never see him again. I think he was just annoyed that I finally walked away from a physically abusive marriage. This decision was not made lightly because as a God-fearing woman I believed in working hard to make my marriage succeed. But when he took all the clothes I owned except what I was wearing; all the photos, personal items and furniture, and threw them in the dumpster outside our apartment, in an effort to teach me a lesson about not coming home when he told me to, I knew I had to leave. That of course is coupled with a lot of physical abuse that I endured regularly. It left the relationship in tatters, but I continued to try to salvage some sort of compromise, especially for my son's sake and my peace of mind.

So I mustered up the courage to take my 7 year old son to the funeral home, thinking it would be good for my Ex to see his son now and to pay my respects. I was right! He was understandably upset and seemed genuinely grateful that we showed up, albeit un-invited. I sat in the rear of the funeral home, and allowed him to take our son to the front row to sit with family. My son was grateful to see his dad, and so I figured I had done something good for them both. After the service, John asked if he could take our son home with him for a few hours. I saw no issue with that and agreed to pick him up at 7pm that evening. That allowed him to have more than 6 hours with his son, and since I did not know how long he would be in town, I thought it was fair.

At 7pm I arrived at the door of his family home. It had been a few years since I was at this house, so memories came flooding back. A woman I did not recognize, answered the door. She was screaming and pointing her finger at me. It took me a minute to try to figure out what she was saying, but eventually I heard, "You're the reason we're fighting, you're the problem!" She kept getting closer and closer to me, and I tried to back up but couldn't move fast enough. Just then my ex-husband came to the door and informed me that he would not be giving me my son back and that I should leave now! Now there were two people screaming at me, and I quickly realized I was in a bad situation. But I was not concerned for myself, I was scared for my son! I thought, if this man has abused me, what would prevent him from doing the same to my son? As he pulled her back into the house, they slammed the door in my face! I didn't get a chance to say anything.

Fear began to consume me, so I ran to my car, and pulled a crowbar from my trunk, I had to get my son out of that house! I ran to the door and banged on it like a crazy woman! "Give me my son!" I screamed so loud it brought the neighbors out of their homes to see what was going on. Now there was a crowd, and tensions where at a point of no return!

When the door opened, there was *that* woman again! She didn't say a word, she just grabbed me and slammed me into the doorway. That was it, I was fighting for my child, and she was in the way! I began to swing, claw, and kick at her. I was wearing false nails and remember scraping them down her face! I was determined to leave my mark! She reciprocated by clawing at me and I quickly realized that she was not as tough as she portrayed. She missed my face with her wild swinging.

Now we were in the house, with a grieving family, everyone was screaming and yelling and trying to pull us apart! Somehow we ended up in the kitchen, and I was on the floor. It was at that moment, that I think my life changed. You see, someone either dropped a microwave on my head or kick me in the head with such force, that I screamed in pain. My insides shook, the room was spinning, and I was totally disoriented! Oh my God, get out of here I thought, "You're alone, YOU, are going to die!" I got up and staggered to the door, I could hear people yelling at me, calling me names and throwing plates, bowls, anything they could get their hands on to hurt me! I was bloody, crying, and afraid! I got to the door in one piece, but I still did not have my son! And that was not going to "fly"! I had to do something. So I jumped in my car and went to get help, the kind of help you wouldn't normally call for, but I was desperate.

Now I have to admit that I did know some seedy characters in the community. And rather than go to the police, my first instinct was to go them for help. I was going to get my son, one way or another. I looked terrible, I was shaking, and honestly felt like I was going to pass out, but my stress level was so high, I was running on adrenaline. I asked my "friend" to give me a gun! I did not care what kind, I just wanted a gun to get my son.

Needless to say, my "friend" tried to calm me down, but he was now upset that someone was hurting me. He sat me in a chair and asked me to tell him what happened as he went to get a first aid kit. I started explaining the situation, while he cleaned my wounds. Re-telling the story made me mad and I got aggravated all over again. He began to bandage the cut on my head. I had to leave now! If he wasn't going to help me, then I had to go…HE GAVE ME THE GUN! I walked out the door, jumped in my car and headed straight back to that house to get my son, one way or the other! What I did not know is that he too got in his car and followed me to the house. He wanted to protect me, and I appreciated that. I pulled up to the house and I left my car in the middle of the street. I got out and headed up the stairs.

I banged on the door again, and this time I was ready. Gun in hand and pointed at the door, I would not let them send me away this time. The door opened but this time it was my ex-husband. He said, 'Why would you come here on this day to fight with my wife?" 'Ahhhh,' I thought to myself that is who she is. I did not bother to reply to his question, I only said, "Give me my son, or you will regret it!" Now he noticed the gun, and said, "Are you kidding me right now?" He stepped back and said he would not give me my son. I then told him that I had called the police and they were coming to execute the warrant for his arrest for non-payment of child support. "I want my son," I reiterated. "NOW!" I yelled it as loud and as angrily as I could.

I could hear my son crying in the background, and it made me more determined to get to him. John walked back to the room where my son was, and brought him to the door. My son ran into my arms. I kept the gun pointed at the door as I went down the stairs backwards. My 'friend" met me at the steps, and said, "Don't worry I got you!" He too had a gun pointed at the door. For some reason I didn't think he had more than one gun, I just knew he had a shady past, one that I only wanted to be acquainted with not involved in. I got to my car and handed him the gun back. I then buckled my son in his seat, locked my doors and drove away. My son never saw his father again until he was 23, and that was by his own choice. I never again spoke to my ex or mentioned his name again.

I tell that story, because I truly believe that the injury to my head, the past beatings, and the stress of the situation helped to bring me to this time. I don't remember much after this. Only that I was constantly looking over my shoulder, trying to protect my son, and give him a life that would minimize the lack of a father. This was a very tough season.

While I do not have a lot of memories of my life, I can still remember that time. That one event, that scarred me, scared me, and just about froze me from living. But God would not have it!

Another memory is of the job I had just before the aneurysm occurred. You see I was Director of Systems Engineering for a Software company in Atlanta. I travelled 3 weeks out of each month and had suitcases lined up in my closet with clothes to grab at any time. One day I would be in France, the next day New York, or London. I saw every state in the US except Nebraska! When I tell you I travelled a lot it would be an understatement.

There was one week that stood out the most! That Monday, I was in New York, and was asked if I would fly to Philadelphia to repair a network that was having issues. Of course I agreed. The company apartment was made ready for my arrival and I flew in that Tuesday morning.

I remember my sister Linda saying, "I'm worried that you're doing too much. You seem tired." I told her I was good and just needed some sleep. I promised I would rest when I got back. I was not really listening, and continued to pack.

I spent 3 days in Philly when I got another call asking me if I could go to Ireland. Well, I had never gone so I was excited, even though I knew I would have to work. Nonetheless I trotted off to Dublin, Ireland where I spent a full week. It was a stressful time because the clients were not cooperating, the computer network was having long delays, and my bosses were looking at me for a miracle. I was tired and stressed, but luckily, I fixed all issues before heading to the airport. My flight to the US was on time and I was grateful. I returned home to Georgia and soon realized that jet-lag was very real and I was really feeling it! By the time I arrived home and got into my apartment, I could barely walk. I fell to my knees as this unbelievable exhaustion came over me. But rather than stopping and resting, I kept pushing a little further. I just needed to be ready for work tomorrow, then I can sleep. My son, now in his twenties, emphatically ordered me to bed as he watched me crawling on the kitchen floor to get a bite to eat. I literally could not walk on my legs. My body had given out on me. As I turned to look at him I hit my head on the cabinet door. I wasn't bleeding just feeling the pain of the impact. My head was now spinning, I need to lie down now! It was a warning sign that I chose to ignore a little longer and a sign I should not have pushed aside.

He said, "I will make you a plate Ma, go to bed!" I did as he said, I had no fight in me, no reasoning left to make a decision. I just needed the bed, NOW! I never ate any food or prepared anything for the next day's work. These events brought me to today.

The next morning at 10:30am, the brain aneurysm ruptured, and I was in trouble!

This was a season of courage.

CHAPTER 2

The day it happened, I remembered I awoke still feeling very tired. But I had to get going, so rest would have to wait. I trotted off to work and I had a one hour drive so, I put on my music and started on my way. I remember thinking how loud the music sounded so I turned it down. That in itself was surprising to me because I love all kinds of music and always played it quite loud, but today it wasn't happening.

So I arrived at work, and said hello to everyone. I was feeling very tired, and was literally dragging myself to my desk. As I sat down, I remember placing a mint in my mouth. At that moment a stabbing pain hit my right eye. Dead center of my eyeball, the pain shot through me. I believe the Annie ruptured at that moment.

I turned and looked at my office mates and told them not to eat the mints I purchased, because they may have sorbitol in them; something I am allergic to. I stood up, threw the mint away, and almost instantaneously, felt nauseous! I started thinking I must be getting sick, so maybe I should go home. I saw my boss in the hallway and told him I was not feeling well and needed to go home. Since I rarely took off, he completely understood. So I pulled out my keys and headed to the parking lot.

That queasy feeling was consuming me and I got to the car, without barfing in the lot. The building has so many windows, that an episode like that could have been embarrassing.

Whew! Finally in the car, I put the key in the ignition, and a massive headache was starting to pound on my right side. Now I'm thinking that I better lay here in the car for a few moments before I take off driving. So I removed my key placed that and my cell phone on the passenger seat and attempted to recline my seat back. OMG!!! Let me say it again, OMG!!! My head went from a low grade headache to the worst pain I have ever had in my life! It felt like someone was swinging a hammer at my head, and they only did it on the right side! I screamed out, "Oh My God, Oh, My God!" Let me push my chair back up and at that exact moment my seat locked upright, I fell forward and slumped on the steering wheel. I think I passed out. The next thing I remember is a young man who was at my car window and he was saying, "Don't worry, we will get you some help!" I remember the horn blowing and it was killing my head. I passed out again.

The next thing I remember is the ambulance drivers saying she may have had a stroke or heart attack. I remember getting mad at that thought, and yelled out I did not have a heart attack! But according to the EMT's and other witnesses my words were slurred an unclear. "She said something, but not making any sense," he said out loud. I passed out again.

The next thing I remember is being air lifted by helicopter to a hospital. The pilot said, "I am going to put headphones on you so you can't hear all the noise." I wanted to say ok, but nothing was working. I hear him say, "She is non-responsive." "Let's move!" How I heard that, I have no idea.

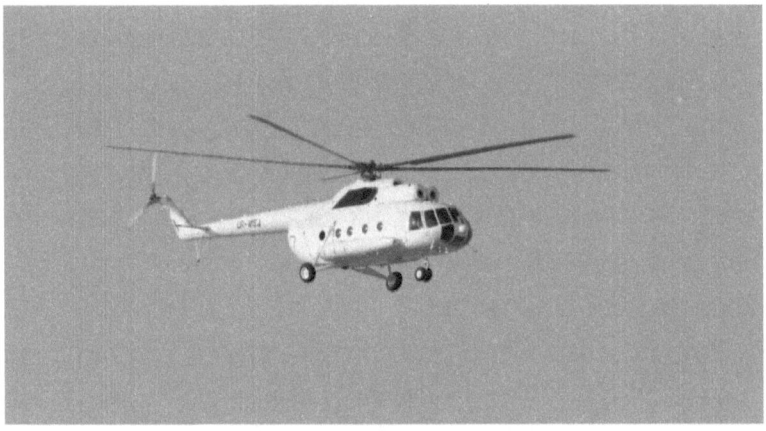

So here you will have to work with me, because everything is just brief images. For example, the Aneurysm occurred on October 28th, I remember that date because I voted early for the Presidential Election. I was unconscious for a few days so I was told. I later found out that the hospital kept me pumped full of morphine. But I do remember hearing my family celebrating in the room, and I opened my eyes briefly to see what was happening? One image remains, the Obama's smiling and walking across a platform. Apparently the Democrats had won the election! The United States had its first African American President, and I was grateful! I lost consciousness again.

I also remember a room with a lot of lights, white in color, and me saying, "I'm alright!" According to the ICU nurse, I woke up during surgery and told the doctors I was ok. I remember someone saying, "Why is she awake? She shouldn't be awake!" Not sure what happened after that. I woke up again 3 months later.

I remember thinking I had taken a much needed nap. I was tired and wanted to sleep, so I did. What I did not know was that I was at the hospital in the intensive care unit. There were plugs coming out of my shaved head, and machines hooked up to every arm, and leg! I was going to get up, and start my day, but my sister Linda, stopped me when she said, "Where are you going Sweetie?" I turned and looked and her and tried to speak, but the words made no sense. I made no sense, she said. Things had changed and I was the only one who did not understand it.

I don't remember much of the rest of the time either at the hospital or at the rehab facility where I stayed another few weeks. I just talked with people and tried to piece together the images I still have with what actually happened.

CHAPTER 3

WHAT NOW?

I can remember after finally getting home with my sister, we sat at the dinner table and I had to panic attack. The fear enveloped me, and for the first time in my life, I was scared, unsure of my next steps! Without thinking, I cried out, "I don't know what to do?" Sherlyn looked at me as if I just hit her with a baseball bat! You see I was always the confident sister, the fearless one, the one who would try almost anything once to see if I could do it! If I enjoyed it I kept doing it! But now, I was lost, and it shook me to my core!

Being a loving and supportive person, she asked, "What do you mean?" Her face was shocked and confused. When she saw my stress, she joined me in the conversation I was obviously having with myself. It wasn't so much what she said, but the way she said it, that made me realize I was walking on thin ice, and she knew it too! I repeated my statement emphatically, "I DON'T KNOW WHAT TO DO!" Tears began to stream down my face.

At that moment she knew she had to lend a hand; to be the caregiver I needed! Sherlyn turned to me and said, "You put one foot in front of the other and you go!" She said it in a warm and quiet voice, because she thought that was the best approach. At that moment I understood I needed help and she was giving it, which I really appreciated. I thought to myself, "What does that mean?" Since the Aneurysm I don't have many feelings about anything. There was a sensation of a plastic bag surrounding my head, and it seemed like that bag was blocking feelings of any kind. It could have also been the prescribed drugs I was taking, and there were many. In the end, I was no closer to figuring things out then I was before my cry for help. Nonetheless, it happened, and I needed answers to so many questions. I had to have more than one sentence to guide me. I had hoped she would have given me a roadmap, a guide something to tell me what to do. There was one specific question that I plagued me to no end. Very simply, it was, "Now what?" "How do I begin to pick up the pieces?" How do I put one foot in front of the other and go?

Oh, I got all the medical advice I could handle, but it was not enough. I needed more. I had the prayers, and family support from everyone for my recovery, but no one had answers for me on what I should do to start living my life again! I had no guidance on how to start the process. I was walking in a fog, it was like literally being born again. Everything was new and I was now this timid person trying to navigate the world!

So, I began looking for my own answers. I began to document what was so clearly not documented for people like me! I started to build my own roadmap for finding a way to deal with this unbelievable situation.

FIRST STEPS

There were plenty of books on brain aneurysms, what were the causes, and even stories of other survivors who made it through. No one wrote or offered advice on how to put one foot in front of the other and go after an Aneurysm! Maybe it was my brain always needing concrete verifiable answers, or maybe it was the anal-retentive behavior I had always exhibited in the past. But it was still lacking for people like me, who needed to know what to expect now; what to do, or how to start? The reality set in, that if I was going to make it, **I had to be the one to create change!** I had to do the work, and it would not be easy.

Everyone was amazed that I had the wherewithal to begin this journey. I mean my speech was impaired, I had difficulty walking without assistance, I could not drive, and was in constant pain. The deck was stacked against me. I had no plan, no ideas on where to go, or where to look. I just knew that CHANGE must happen, if I was going to be successful…and make no mistake, I was going to be successful, I would have to be determined! I was always a go getter, and this was the season of exploration! Time to get busy.

Before we begin this, let me tell you what this book is not. It is not some medical journal on the causes of an aneurysm; it is also not a book about my journey, although I do reference some of my personal experiences along with others! It's also not the "feel sorry for me," book, although I do hope you walk away with some empathy, and a better understanding for aneurysms and the havoc they can cause.

What I hope is that this book will make every survivor and caregiver have a place to begin; a starting point for what happens to each of us **after** this episode. By expounding on life for an "Annie" (Aneurysm) survivor who does not have obvious signs or deformities as a result of this event.

If you are lucky or blessed enough to live to talk about it, I hope this book will help. This is a story of what we feel and experience, and how to help us to get started! A simple and honest account of what daily life is like! Please know I am offering advice and real world examples of what I have researched and lived through. I am by no means an expert, just a conscientious survivor who wanted to make a difference.

I wrote this to help others understand our situation and to help survivors know you are not alone. You are not imagining things or being overly dramatic. The experiences you now have are real! They will not define you, but they do let you know that you must take an alternate path.

Let me tell you plainly, the person you knew is gone, you are different now! You will never be the same! But you can expect things to get better with time. This book will help you know the seasons you maybe in and how to cope! Using some of the things written here can help you navigate this murky world in which you now live. There are phases that bring excitement and others that make you wonder how are you going to get through it? But you WILL get through it, I promise!

One thing you have to remember is that life is about seasons. Seasons where you go through ups and downs, good and bad. As I say that, it is not to reveal some major commentary on life, but to draw a stark contrast into what Annie survivors go through. Our seasons are more intense, more intricate in what others take as everyday circumstance. To an Annie survivor, let me state that our seasons are anything but a common occurrence.

In the beginning you have to know that this is the season of adjustment. Learning how to navigate the new world you now live with. If you're like me, and in your early 50s, you may have to re-learn everything. Your body has changed, and your thoughts are not clear. Processing any information is slower, and physical movement is now a daunting task of muscle memory and execution. You will find methods of adjustment and conditions when nothing you put in place works. But know that you must keep going, you must hold on to the truth that this season will pass.

CHAPTER 4

NOW LET'S GET STARTED

As I scoured the internet looking for information; a book, a blog, or anything that would shed some light on what has happened; what I was feeling, I found no written material. I checked all the major books sights and I even talked with hospitals in different cities. I joined support groups and even wandered into hypnosis for context. I wanted a guide for my new life, so I googled every term or diagnosis I uncovered. Somebody had to have some information they could share?

Instead, I quickly discovered that I could read a ton of medical journals, which I could not understand clearly. I could talk to people who simply thought I should just get on with my life, or I could just float in the blind knowledge that there were few survivors, so the available materials are lacking. I could not believe there was nothing out there that could help me deal with life now? I have talked to doctors and hospitals, fellow survivors and even my Pastor, but no one could relate to the world I now lived in. Oh, they did offer great empathy, but unless you lived through this you cannot fully understand. Why is it so taboo talk about how to survive now? I knew I had to have answers but where to find them? I was left with little to nothing. So, I began this journey of enlightenment for myself and for others like me. I documented everything that was happening, everything that I couldn't explain. I asked a ton of questions. I asked so many questions that I am sure I got on everyone's nerves! But with that, I was now fully armed and ready for battle. And make no mistake, this is a battle! My hope is that this book will offer you, me, and our caregivers the opportunity to see clearly who we have become, and how to go upward from here. It took me 10 years and a nagging push from God, to know that I must write this book, to help myself and other survivors as well as the friends and family of survivors to understand. If you remember nothing else about this book know this, 'CHANGE HAS COME!' The person you knew has undergone a life altering metamorphosis and has come out the other side!

I often think about how long it took for the world to embrace the Special Needs community, and the delicate processes which had to be adopted when working or living with them. I want this book to start the conversation about Aneurysms and Annie survivors!

No this is not the 'woe is me' story, instead it is a look at the strength it takes daily for a survivor! How amazing life can be when we really understand the issues we face! Here are the answers you wanted to get but could not find or were afraid to ask.

This book will help survivors understand that our world now at times can be introverted, painful, and even sluggish. It will allow you to relate to what we live with daily. It may even open the conversation for new discussions between the survivor and the caretakers. TALK! It will help! I pray you learn what I have discovered, we are a special class and we are weaker but not powerless!

FIRST THINGS FIRST – A SUPPORT SYSTEM

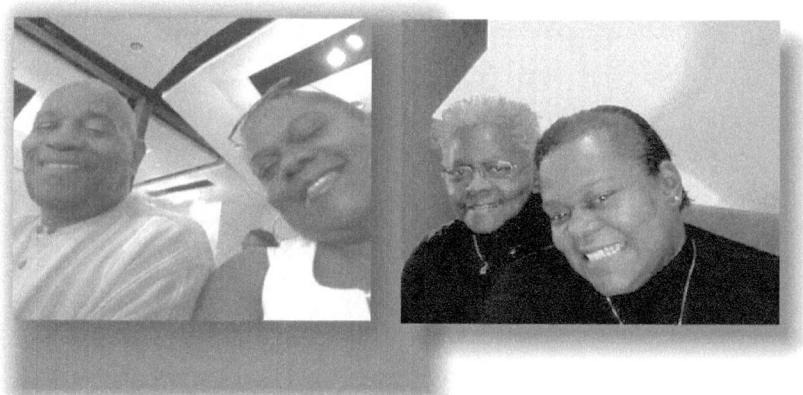

This is my Mom and Dad, my rocks! As you can see, the right side of my head was shaved from surgery, and one eye is partially damaged. That is because my Annie was on that side behind my right eye, and yes, I had a craniotomy (a surgical operation in which a bone flap is temporarily removed from the skull to access the brain.) The Annie was coiled so, I live with the fact that it could rupture again at any moment! I still have a great deal of difficulties seeing on that side or even walking, but that smile says it all...I made it! My Mom bathed me when I couldn't do it for myself, she fed me when I couldn't feed myself! She monitored my meds when I forgot to take one of the many pills I was prescribed. After finally leaving the physical therapy facility and getting back home, she made me smile for the camera! She reminded me that I am still here! My Dad always has a funny story to uplift me or some scripture to guide me! She and my Dad are amazing! Because of their love, the love of my 3 incredible sisters, my unbelievably strong son, daughter-in-law, and my loving grandkids, my best friend Debra, I persevere! They are my support team!

If you're wondering where to *start*, then the first thing you need to do is get a *support team* if you don't already have one. It could be someone new or a tried and true family member, just build a support team. Let them know the role you need them to play. One of my sisters, is my encouragement guru. She lifts me when I feel down, and all I have to do is call or text and she comes running. There is also my prayer buddy, who when I feel lost, offers prayers, nothing more, just prayers! I even have a comedian friend who makes me laugh. His jokes are always needed and come even when I don't ask. I also enlisted a *tears* buddy, someone who lets me cry on those days that I need to release the overwhelming sadness I feel. She does not judge, she just says, "Let it out, it's ok I'm here!" My son handles my healthcare and monitors how much I exert myself daily. He sees what I sometimes miss. My daughter-in-law is my monitor. She does all those superwoman things I can no longer do. She is the mother of the greatest grandkids in the world! They are smart, funny, helpful, and full of energy. Just what a Grandmother needs! These are just a few of the team members of my support system. I have too many to name, but they know who they are and the roles they play.

I want to let you know that a *support system* is crucial in this fight. It can be your family, friends, a community group, your Pastor or Priest, or even a doctor! These are the people you can lean on when there are good or bad days. Whomever you choose, keep them on speed dial. Let them know that you need to depend on them from time to time to support your recovery efforts.

Make sure they understand the purpose of your support team and their new role in your life. Be honest about the type of help you need. This is the season of building, so build strategically.

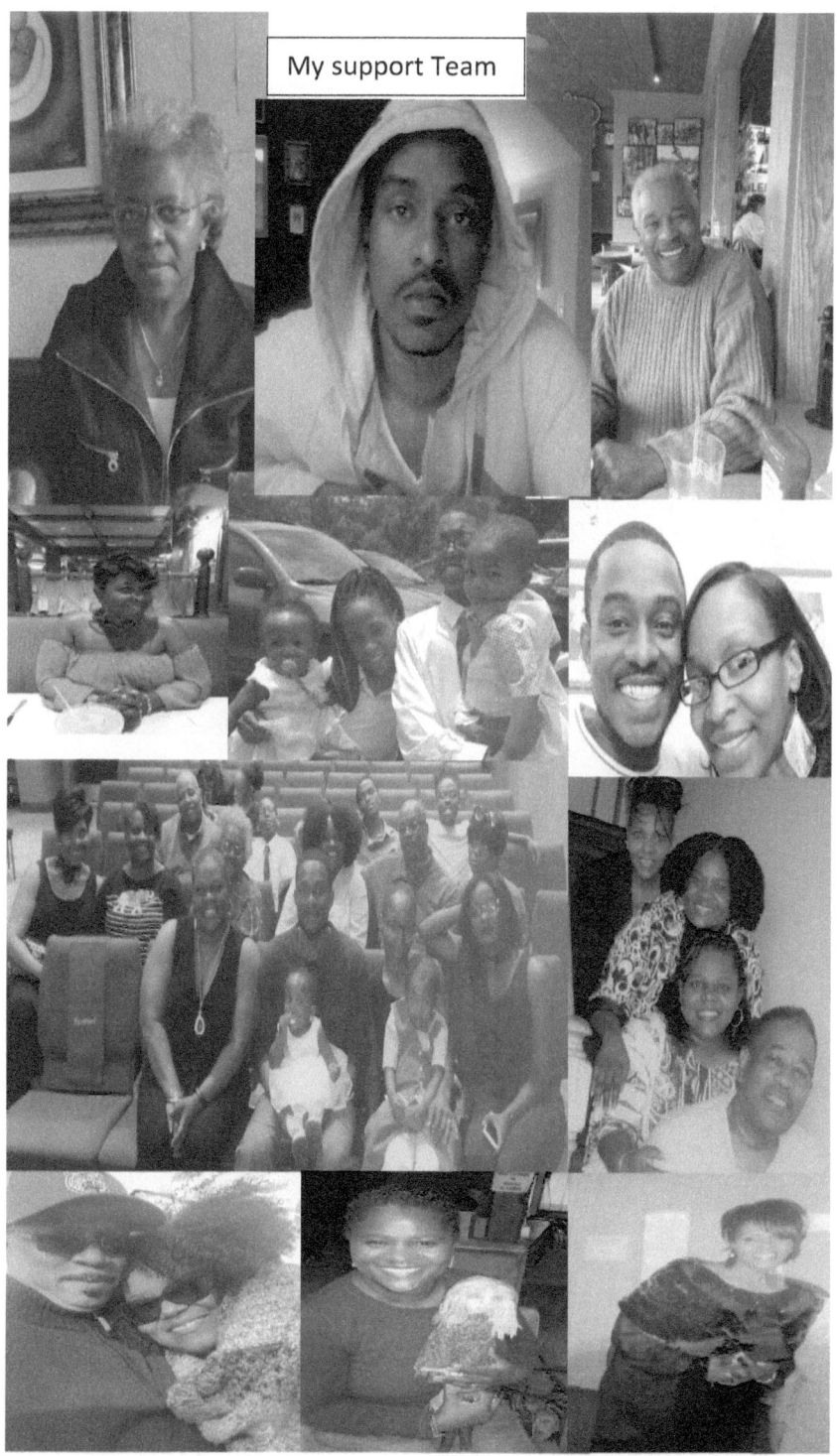

CHAPTER 5

COMMUNICATION ROLES

For the caregiver, whomever you are to the Survivor, know that you play an **extremely important** role to us. You are our leaning post, the one true constant in this new world we live in! This is for you to know that what you are doing is selfless, supportive, and greatly appreciated!

If I can offer one piece of advice to the support team: talk with others in the group. I found out very quickly that making sure all the group members know what may be happening is critical to our success. This is because you may be able to pick up on things that are happening and can then collaborate on a plan for moving our focus along or getting medical attention if needed. Remember that you are not only our leaning post, but also a guide that we trust most to walk with us through this intimidating journey. Remember that life as we knew it is over, and we are unsure of everything. You were chosen for just such a time as this! Please continue to be present and observant.

MEDICATIONS

Ok I have to address this because I was also placed on a plethora of meds that helped in some cases but caused adverse reactions in other cases.

You, the Annie survivor, must talk about how you feel when you take your meds! You must share with your doctors and support team the issues these meds present. Now, I am not suggesting you get off your meds or take more of them, what *I am recommending is that you watch, document, and relay what you feel.* It is crucial to your success.

I can remember one of the pills my first Neuro Surgeon prescribed. It caused hemorrhoids and severe constipation so badly that I thought I would die from the pain. I shared that info with the doctor, but he thought I should try to do things like a sitz bath, or drink more water. He explained it was really crucial that I take this pill so try to make it work. I was in tears each time I had to use the restroom. There was a rash on my arms and my breathing was becoming labored. I even developed what I call the 'Harlem shake," actually it was a very pronounced tremor over my entire body. So, I suffered a few more weeks, until I could not take it anymore. I did not know what else I could do, so I went to get help. I called my sister in tears begging for help. She gathered the support team and began getting things under control.

My Mom made an appointment with the doctor and after admittance to the hospital, my sister advocating for me, and a thorough exam, this team of doctors determined that I was having an allergic reaction and immediately took me off the meds. It took some convincing of this team of psychologist that is was not in my head, or some type of PTSD. They prescribed a different medication and I began to feel better shortly. I am allergic to everything so I have to be careful what I take. My support team was crucial in helping me get through this. I shared that story because it was just one of the many issues you could face if you do not watch your meds. Be your own health advocate. Talk to anyone and everyone when you don't feel right, it could just be the meds you are taking.

Needless to say, I no longer have this doctor, because if you are not going to listen and trust that I know what feels right or wrong with my body, then I can no longer work with you. I could have ended that suffering weeks earlier.

DOCTORS

I now have an amazing Interventional Neuro Radiologists, Spine Specialists, and a Primary Care Physician who listen and welcome my input with the health plan we are implementing. They have gotten me off multiple medications and applaud my efforts with physical therapy. They have repaired my spine, adjusted prescriptions, and monitor my health from a total body perspective. Finally I have a, PCP, although new to my health team, she and my other doctors are some of the most dynamic, caring woman doctors I have ever met! They actually want to get to know me, not just medicate me, and that is priceless! They all know how important it is to re-gain my independence! They help me to remain patient in my recovery and do all that they can to help me succeed.

Knowing and choosing your doctors is extremely important. Don't just accept a doctor because they were there when you woke up. Do they listen to your concerns, or is it lip service? Do they want you to improve and ultimately migrate off of any meds when appropriate or medically sound to do so? Are they asking the right questions about being an Annie survivor? Do YOU take any of your support team with you to appointments? They can help assess the doctor and give you good feedback in your decision making process.

Whatever your process and whomever your doctor(s) know that you have to be present to work with them. You have to write down concerns, talk with them about issues, and work together to be a better person. Find a way to get to that good place, and know this is the season of Advocating for yourself!

CHAPTER 6

GOOD DAYS BAD DAYS

This is a pretty simple topic, and one that I think anyone who has survived a catastrophic illness can relate to. We have good days and bad days. There is no rhyme or reason as to what will constitute either, but there is the fact that you can quickly recognize it.

What makes a good day? Waking up! Sometimes we survivors forget to remember the small things, such as seeing one more day! We miss the forest for the trees, so to speak.

That is where you, the support team comes in, because we can get so lost in the minutia of daily activities that we forget to stop and realize the blessings. Yes, it may be difficult, or we may process information slower today, but it IS! Help us to remember that; to see the good in all the things that we have done that others may not get to do! Remember this simple fact, there are few survivors of a ruptured Brain Aneurysm!

For me a good day was waking up with no pain...a rare occasion...but it has happened. My family is instrumental in helping me cope with the pain when I would forget how to do that! There is nothing more aggravating than having to reach for a pain pill first thing in the morning.

Other survivors have talked about a good day for them, meant taking a walk to see the sun, or dressing themselves. Any little thing is a time of celebration for an Annie survivor. Let us celebrate the things we accomplish, because it is truly a wonderful feat for us! Join in by offering accolades to yourself for something you accomplished, you deserve it too! It will empower the feeling of moving forward; of improvement.

Now for the bad days. Let's be honest, just about anything can be the culprit for a bad day. That is when it is most important for your support team to breakout understanding and patience. We are lost sometimes and bringing us out of this funk can do wonders for the survivor and the caregiver! But it must be done with patience, because we will go kicking and screaming into a new level of bad day, without that support.

I remember having one of those bad days early in my recovery. I was extremely emotional with tears flowing like a river, and could not figure out how to stop it. I hated the fact that I was an in-patient in a physical therapy facility. I was mad at the world that I could not walk and needed a wheel chair! My sister Kim would call every morning and sing a song of encouragement over the phone. As a gospel singer, she knows how to encourage others through music, but on this day, it did not help. The last thing I wanted was a song. I wanted to go home!

Stubborn as she is, she would not hang up until she found a way to reach me. I realized quickly if I did not pull myself together should would not leave me alone. So, I began to muster the courage to follow her into the light of happiness she so willingly shared with me. It was contagious, and I began to believe again that I would be ok. My pain became manageable with the help of pain meds and some faith. My Bad day diminished with her help!

A short time later my son arrived, and I could see the fear in his eyes, as he saw me struggling to speak clearly, and that I would never be whole again. He tried to cover it up, but it was written all over his face. Since I was his only parent, his heart was broken for the suffering I was going through. Being a parent helps in finding strength you never thought you had, and I did not want him to worry, or feel afraid any longer. So, I worked harder, to show him I would not give up and neither should he!

Bad days can cause blood pressures to rise, increase the strength of a headache, or even slur speech. Bad days can also keep us in bed for days at a time! I actually spent more than 2 days in bed, because I just didn't feel well. I had no energy, no desire to function, so I laid there like a bump on a log. On the third day, my support team intervened and began focusing on issues I did not realize were affecting me. You see, we actually had a week of rain and it was causing low grade headaches, but I tried to tough it out instead of saying, "I hurt." This moment of bad days can consume us and that is where you come in. You need to bring us out, help us be stronger with gentle patience and loving kindness. Offer a medication fix, or a walk outside. Whatever it is that is needed; or will help is what your support team must accomplish.

I would like to tell you Caregivers it will be easy, but it will not. Many times we are lost on how to fix things; or how to get back to a level place, but you must figure it out for us.

Remember that while you're helping your survivor, how do you help yourself? Find time to care for you, and to be grateful that you are able to help. Listen to a favorite song, or just have a cup of tea on the porch for 5 minutes…you must take care of yourself as well. Although we may not say it often enough, please know we see your efforts, and we *really* appreciate you. These things will help you to continue to help us, I promise.

As I was writing this chapter, I had one of those dreaded bad days. It all began with a trip to a new doctor. The office was located in a city I was unfamiliar with. Instead of me doing my normal routine of getting the address and confirming the time I needed to arrive. I waited until the day of the appointment to plan my route. BIG MISTAKE!! Now of course you'd think that I have GPS so I could have put the address in the system and would have had no issues. But here was the problem; I googled the Doctor and chose an old address which they had moved from. I did not know that. So I started off to my intended destination and arrived with 15 minutes to spare! I was proud of myself, time to celebrate a little. I accomplished this on my own! When I walked in and could not find the Doctor on the directory board, I quickly realized it must be the wrong address! I could feel the panic setting in, as I called the office for the correct address. The receptionist informed that they had moved from this location more than a year ago...and they were now located more than 20 minutes away. Now I was in a full-on panic, because I would not be able to make it to the appointment in time. But the receptionist said, "Give it a try we'll do our best to hold your place." So off I went, and after a few wrong turns, and 45 minutes of traffic I finally arrived. I tried to walk in the office and hoped all would be ok. But for an Annie survivor, it is not the case. Any deviation in our plans, can throw us off our game. It stresses us out and highlights the deficits we now live with. You see I was now on a hospital campus and had to park far away from the doctor's office. I saw a ton of buildings and none had the correct address. I am now roaming the campus lost and seconds from losing total control. So once again I called the doctor's office and now in tears, and 30 minutes late, I relay the fact that I cannot find their office and I need help! The receptionist thank God was a kind woman and began to guide me step-by-step to her office from where I was standing. I finally arrived and was obviously in distress. The asked me to sit, got me a glass of water and then tried to salvage the appointment. I began to calm down, but it was useless, I was devastated by my mistake.

Unfortunately, the doctor had an emergency at the hospital and could not see me. That one statement broke me down. I was so frustrated with myself for not doing what needed to be done to prevent this situation, that I could not fight back my tears. So we rescheduled my appointment and I headed back to my car. I was so sad, so afraid because my mind had gone blank. I had stressed myself out so much that I could not figure out how to get home. I called all my support team members, and like any 'perfect storm', no one answered their phones. This made me even more stressed out and afraid of what I to do next! Then I pulled over on the shoulder of the highway and began to pray for guidance. I needed help now. My phone and my GPS were readily available, but for the life of me I could not figure out what to do or how to use them. It was like being in a pitch-dark room and feeling your way around, only to realize you can't find anything. You don't even recognize anything. My tears started to flow again, I WAS SCARED! For the first time in a long time, I had a reminder of the problems I still face, and what can go terribly wrong if I get lost.

Thank God, I got help...a tiny voice said, 'try again.' So I called my Mom first this time, and she answered! She heard my fear, and started the process we implemented to help me get back to control. As a survivor you will always have times when the world does not make sense, and you're lost as to what to do. Needless to say, I plan and pre-plan, even the most-minute details now...it helps, trust me!

This was a season of learning to properly plan all activities.

CHAPTER 7

My wall of organization

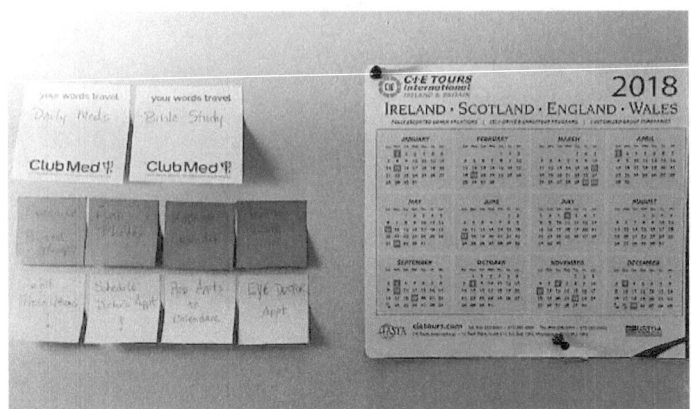

DAILY LIVING

We all have our daily routines, the things we do as if on auto pilot. Things like brushing your teeth, washing your face, or combing your hair. For an aneurysm survivor that daily routine is crucial to our existence. As is evidenced by the photo above. For some of us we have a million sticky notes in various colors so that we could organize our daily routine. My wall contains the orange sticky for my important notes like appointments, with doctors, the blues are things to remember like updating the calendar, and the white are must complete everyday items. It took me several years to figure out how I would be able to remember so many things. Remember that we are new to everything and we have to figure out what to do. That is where our support system comes into play. We may forget to add a reminder. You will have to be our memory and yours as well. But keep this in mind, while it may be a little daunting now, we will get better and get to point to where we will not need the help. BUT that is not going to happen right away.

We want to feel the pride in remembering the things that so many of us take for granted. So how do we get through this season? Very simply; get a plan that works, whether it be sticky pads, notebooks, your phone a phone call from a friend. Just create a plan that will help you get your independence back. And yes, I know that is the one thing that affects every survivor, is the fact that we are now dependent on others! Trust me I get it, but also know that if you are patience and practice daily routines, you will get through this. Take it easy on your support team, they too are trying to navigate this new reality just like you. Sometimes I can literally walk into the kitchen to get something to eat, and the time it took to get from the bedroom to the kitchen; I completely forgot what was I going to do? Now many people will say they do that as well and have not suffered from an Annie, but let me tell you it is completely different for us. We suffer from significant short-term memory loss. Let me tell you that most survivors are the same, and no this is not old age or forgetfulness, this is one of the components of an Annie. My friend Allen, also a survivor, suffers as well from short term memory loss. He often forgets when he is driving, where he is going and has had to pull over and start again to his desired destination. Lately, he has given up driving, unless absolutely necessary. That is when the GPS comes in handy, if you remember to put in the correct address of a destination!

For most Aneurysm patients it is a real accomplishment to remember anything. I find myself using sticky pads in order of operation, so I don't miss a step. My IPhone has a great feature where I can setup reminders, it has proven very helpful in that regard.

I remember I was baking chocolate chip cookies for my grandkids, and forgot the chips. What I should have done, was taken all my ingredients out of the pantry and then I would have seen them. But I didn't, and my grandkids quickly mentioned what I forgot. I was disappointed, and I felt frustration with myself for forgetting something so important to good chocolate chip cookies. My grandkids quickly told me that it was ok, and we ate them anyway! Forgetting routine steps is just one of the many ways our daily living has been altered by what has happened.

Mary, another survivor, told me she was headed out the door to church when she realized she had forgotten to put on shoes. When the cold of the porch touched her feet, she stopped and thought how silly she was to forget something so simple. But when she went back into the house, she also forgot what she came back for? She is reminded often of the changes in her daily living and she is only 24 years old!

I have even forgotten my point when speaking; right in the middle of a conversation!

When you see us looking lost or unsure of what should be happening next, give us a helping hand. A lot of times, we are too ashamed to ask for help, or too afraid to admit we don't know. But don't treat us like children. We simply need a little help, not hand holding. The short-term memory loss affects our daily living processes in such a way as to be one of the key elements most of our caregivers miss. We look normal, we talk pretty good most of the time, but it is a daily struggle.

This is the season of acceptance!

CHAPTER 8

THE WHY AND THE WHY ME PHASE?

Ok, so I need to take a moment to touch this stage, because it lends credence to what has happened to survivors.

There is a point in the recovery stage where we begin to ask why? What did we do to have this happen to us? What was it about me that caused such trauma? I can tell you that I often asked that question, as have many other Annie survivors. Especially since I didn't have any warning. I had no diabetes, or high blood pressure, cancer, or even a bad tooth? There was no rhyme or reason, it just happened. Yes it could have been stress or the physical abuse I suffered, but I will never know. It took most of the past 10 years to come to terms with this fact.

Most Annie survivors feel the same. What did we do to cause this issue? The reality is that this was most likely a hereditary trait. There are some doctors who think most Aneurysm lie dormant for years in all of us, and then one day they rupture. We've all had family members who experienced a ruptured aneurysm, but maybe at that time it was not correctly diagnosed. Or they passed away suddenly and without symptoms. Could it have been an Aneurysm?

The fact is that doctors are still learning about Aneurysm and much more info needs to be discovered and shared with the world. Survivors of a ruptured Annie and rare and can offer the medical community a closer look as to what happens *after* the rupture. They should reach out and do some studies to help in their quest for understanding of this medical phenomenon. It has got to be more than a questionnaire with little to no regard for what life is like now! The research MUST include the life after an Annie! It has changed us, redirected our paths and made us look toward what we can do now with what we have. It cannot be what society says it should be, but instead what we can offer and what society must accept!

The reality is we don't know why because each of us has had something that caused it, and everyone is different. So, asking, "Why me?" is a moot point that can never be fully answered or understood.

This was a season of understanding.

CHAPTER 9

CONSTRUCTION UNDER WAY 39

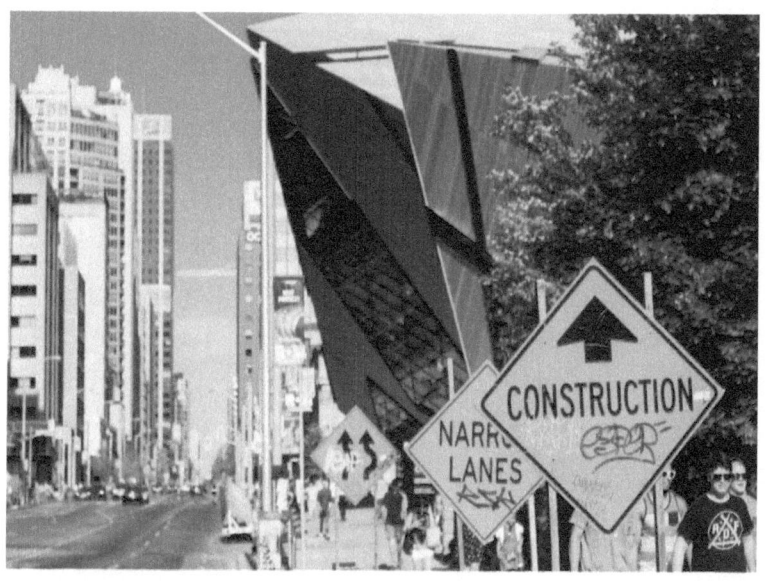

BE PATIENT THINGS ARE HAPPENING!

PHYSICAL THERAPY

I would love to tell you that this was my favorite part of recovery, but it wasn't. It is painful, it was hard, and it was tiring! I remember the 1st week at the physical therapy center, I had no control of my body. I had a wheelchair and a walker. My bladder had a mind of its own, but I could always trust that every 20 minutes or, so I had to go. It was frustrating to need assistance and while waiting for help to go to the bathroom; lying in my bed, I was now a wet mess. I cried when my sister and nurse both arrived to help, and had to admit in my broken communication, that I needed to be changed. Needless to say, their faces provided proof that they were sorry they did not come sooner. It was so humiliating!

It was at that moment that I began to fight for my strength! I knew I could not go through that again, so I worked hard, every day with the team who would help me learn to walk, talk, and care for myself again! It was the hardest thing I have ever done! I wished I could say I never had that soiling incident again, but I can't. It took a lot of courage to admit this, but it was a long while before I had some control over my body. I often wonder what people expect of survivors when it comes bodily functions? I never even gave it a thought, until it happened to me, multiple times!

My PT Nurse was so caring and understanding, and she offered me this advice, "It's only for a season!" With that one statement, I felt like God picked me up and was carrying me through this journey. That nurse had no idea the impact she made on me at that moment! She had no idea that I would be encouraged by her words. I will always be grateful for her.

My Pastor once said that, "You never know how your ministry may help someone else!" He was right. I wanted to write this book because I hoped my journey, my words would encourage someone else. In the season of life, you have to choose to fight, choose to win, choose to succeed, but most of all you have to choose to live!

Every Annie survivor has the same type of story. The one person that took them from sad and afraid to hopeful and determined. It is only for a season and you have to believe you can get through it.

I still have to do physical therapy. I wish I could say I was done, but the reality is I will ever be done. Although I don't go daily anymore, I MUST still do it to keep my muscles working properly! I still take meds and have continual doctor appointments, but I am ok with that. I sometimes hate PT, but I know the short term pain will keep me moving, and that is the ultimate goal.

This is a season of determination and hard work!

CHAPTER 10

THE HEADACHE

Every Annie survivor lives with one fact, one constant: and that is, 'The Headache.' We all live with a constant headache that we must manage daily. It is always sitting in the background, throbbing and waiting for a chance to explode with full force! I wish I could say, that some don't have to deal with this, but the truth is, all survivors are left with it! The question is to what severity will it hurt?

There are many causes to the dreaded headache, most survivors know the triggers. For example, sudden or sever weather changes can cause a headache. Sleep patterns can also cause headaches, a rough night of pain, poor pillow placement, or just lack of sleep can ensure you will wake with a headache. Things like impending rain or snow showers are big culprits. Any weather-related changes can add to the level of pain we feel. Lights in the bedroom from a clock/cable box or TV can also severely increase that headache pain. Light sensitivity is a big culprit for brain aneurysm survivors.

Finally, the most obvious factor for a bad headache is stress! If we do not do all that we can to de-stress our lives and our environment, we are surely in for a rough patch of headaches. It is a requirement that survivors stay as stress free as possible. Try to recognize, when we may not, that we are under stress and need a little help.

It is imperative that we keep control of the headache. Most survivors will take some prescription or over the counter medications to keep it under control. Others will try more holistic methods such as aromatherapy or acupuncture, or even medical marijuana. I found that in my little world the thought of taking too many pills was not an option. So, I began doing simple things like making sure the room is completely dark at bedtime. I also have about 10 pillows to place under my head, legs, or neck when I toss and turn throughout the night.

On those nights when I really can't handle it alone, I will reach for some type of medication, and unfortunately that has become more frequent than I would like. Still others may just turn on the radio with some smooth jazz. Whatever the choice, control is the definite end-game. Figure out your needs and your methods of alleviation and do something about it!

This is the season of mitigation!

THE PAIN

Let me first say this is real! There are days when we experience pain that we cannot explain. Because this cannot be labeled as chronic due to the varying locations, times, and durations, it just is painful. Some survivors have had multiple angiograms, (a specialized X-ray used to look at your veins), and as a result pain can be felt in the groin area. Lower back pains, neck pains, and even eye or ear pain. All I can say is that there is pain, daily!

As a caregiver, remember that we are at our weakest when we are in pain. Why? It is a reminder that our body was traumatized, and our strength is focused on one thing, ENDING THE PAIN!

Allen, told me that when he is pain, he must go to bed, nothing else will work. I try to push through my pain and end up walking with a cane and a limp. It forces my body to curl up like elderly person with spinal problems. As a caregiver, you must understand that we can't stop the pain from happening, and we may suffer a little more than most because of all the things our body has gone through.

Most Annie survivors can even predict the rain! Mary told me she can tell a few days before if bad weather is coming. Jonathan said he has a constant pain in his neck, and is something he cannot understand since his rupture was repaired with a clip. He thought he would be immune to the pain.

Every survivor lives with some sort of pain and every survivor has their own pain threshold. That line in the sand that says, 'I hurt and I need it to stop, NOW!'

Your job as the caregiver is to recognize that we are in pain and try to help us find some way of relieving it. Honestly, because we live with it daily we may not even realize how bad it has become until it is too late. All we know is that we are not feeling good, but we must go through the list of options as to what the cause could be. Sometimes you can look at our face, and determine that pain is happening, and get us through it!

This is the season of diminishing pain.

THE EXHAUSTION

One of the most annoying things for most Annie survivors is the exhaustion that comes on so quickly and with little to no exertion. A simple walk, a long ride in the car can result in exhaustion. I find it quite amazing that taking a very large multivitamin and a B12 pill do little to nothing for the level of exhaustion I feel regularly.

"It is hard to explain," says my friend Allen. "You can sleep 8 hours and wake up to your morning routine, but by the time you're done, your tired and need to rest!" I find it also very true that I tire easily. Even with physical therapy 3 times a week! The lack of energy can also stop us from doing as much as we want, which can be very frustrating.

So, what can you do about the exhaustion? I'm afraid not much. Your body is still sending you warning signals. Take the exhaustion as a sign that you are still healing, and rest is the best method to alleviate these feelings.

This is the season of restful recovery.

CHAPTER 11

I HEAR YOU!

This chapter is for the Annie Survivor alone! I hear you, I understand your pain, your exhaustion, your headaches, and most of all your fears! I understand what you want most at this point in your life. You want to be heard, to be related to, and without hesitation you want to feel accepted!

Let me say it again, I hear you! I walk with the same thoughts of life that you do. I can say that because I have been where you are now. You need to find some light in all this darkness. Well let me tell you that there is light; a light that only we survivors can see and feel. Writing this book has helped me to know one thing. I had work to do! I had a story to tell, to anyone who would listen. I had to put on paper what had been hidden in my mind for 10 years! I had to share the thoughts that plague me weekly, and daily, even hourly. At different times, my thoughts wandered to what can I do now, that I am disabled? Who am I supposed to be, and what do people expect of me? Can I meet those expectations?

The answer is simple, you are what YOU say or want to be from this moment on! Think of it as new beginning, a chance to change the way you think and feel. The start of the best days of your life. In other words, you are a unique and dynamic person who has only one thing to focus on, and that is YOU! The person you become is what you want to be. I find that the stressed out, angry person I used to be is no longer acceptable. I got a second chance to do something different, something better! And now you can too! Don't let this thing that has happened to you break your will. Don't let it define you. Know that everything you are feeling is real, but it does not end here! Find ways to make it better for yourself. Look for excitement, even if it is just dressing yourself daily! Do it in the most helpful and happy way you can! See the joy in reaching a new level each day. Take tiny steps, small goals that help to grow your confidence.

Life is different, but no less exciting and fun! Change the way you view your life and watch how it changes for you! Don't be afraid to say how you feel and embrace the new you, I promise, you will be amazed at the success you find.

CHAPTER 12

BRAIN FOG

There is a dark room with nothing but a file cabinet in it. In the file cabinet are all the memories, thoughts, photos, or anything else you carry in your mind at any given time. When you need to remember a name, or remind yourself of a memory you can go to that file cabinet and retrieve it. Unless you had a Brain Aneurysm, then that file cabinet seems a million miles away! No matter how much you run into that dark room and look for a light, you cannot find one! You can hear the echo in your mind and quickly realize that you can't remember a thing...I always image someone running up a stair case and all you hear is the tap of their shoes with each step. Nothing else is going on...but that noise in your head.

That is what it is like for an Annie survivor. The lights are not working properly, and we must find our way slowly. Yes, you can tell us something you remember so vividly that it seems obvious that we would remember, but the truth is we don't.

My reality set in when I could not remember the first 4 years of my son's life. I can remember images that flash like photos in my head, but they don't always make sense. To me they are just flashes and I cannot tell you what they mean. People often don't believe the level of damage that I have sustained, but do try to help.

Melissa, another survivor says she has lost most of her memory before the Annie. She is sometimes sad when others recount tales of their past and all she has is the days in the hospital and physical therapy center. I remind her that she has the chance to make new memories and sometimes it helps. But the reality is, it frustrates her and me as well.

Allen says his memory is like a funnel. Somethings get through and some don't. As he is more than 10 years out from his Annie, he says his memory has not gotten better over time. My advice, be patient with yourself, because everyone is different. You never know what will come back if you give your brain time to heal!

This is something that is critical to make happen. I know that I have had to rely on others to fill in the memory gaps I now have. My sister Sherlyn, will offer photos, stories, and reading material to help me remember the things that were lost. I can only explain the memory loss the way Dianna, a fellow survivor from my support group, shared with me. She said it's like a hole that is deep and wide and you cannot find the bottom no matter how hard you look. It is just a hole, nothing more, nothing less.

Hmmm...I don't know what season this is...just try to get through it.
SLEEP DEPRIVED

Now this something that I must pass on to you the survivor and the care giver! I will say it plainly, **we do not sleep without some type of sleep aid!** That is the reality we live with daily.

Just like you, we Annie survivors can stay awake all night. Even if we are exhausted, there is no sleep without help.

When I first got out of rehab, I told the doctors how I would be up all night, desperate for sleep, but not able to relax enough to close my eyes. I would try everything including a bath with lavender, chamomile tea, warm milk, or a bedside aroma therapy waterfall. Nothing would help. My doctor offered what so many others do, a prescription sleep aid.

Now I am not opposed to those who take them, you have to do what is best for you. But I can tell you that I was afraid of taking too many pills. Especially those pills that keep you from remembering what you did last night, or the cost of yet another prescription!

So I opted for a simpler approach, one that worked for me. I chose an over the counter pain pill with a sleep-aid in it. Now please realize I am not recommending anything. I did my research and I talked with my doctor, so please do the same thing before you take anything. You are fragile now and you can't do things willy-nilly. But my choice did help with getting the quality sleep I needed to function daily. The importance of sleep cannot be overstated for Annie survivors. Allen refuses to take any pills, he tries to calm his mind and sleeps when he can. If that would work for me, I would be ok, but sadly that is not the case.

Funny thing almost every Annie Survivor I have spoken with states the same thing, that they have difficulty sleeping. We know it is a result of the Annie, but my goodness, a little heads-up that it could happen would have been nice to know. I spent many a night thinking I was depressed and not that there could be a chemical imbalance.

This is the season of finding your way.

CHAPTER 13

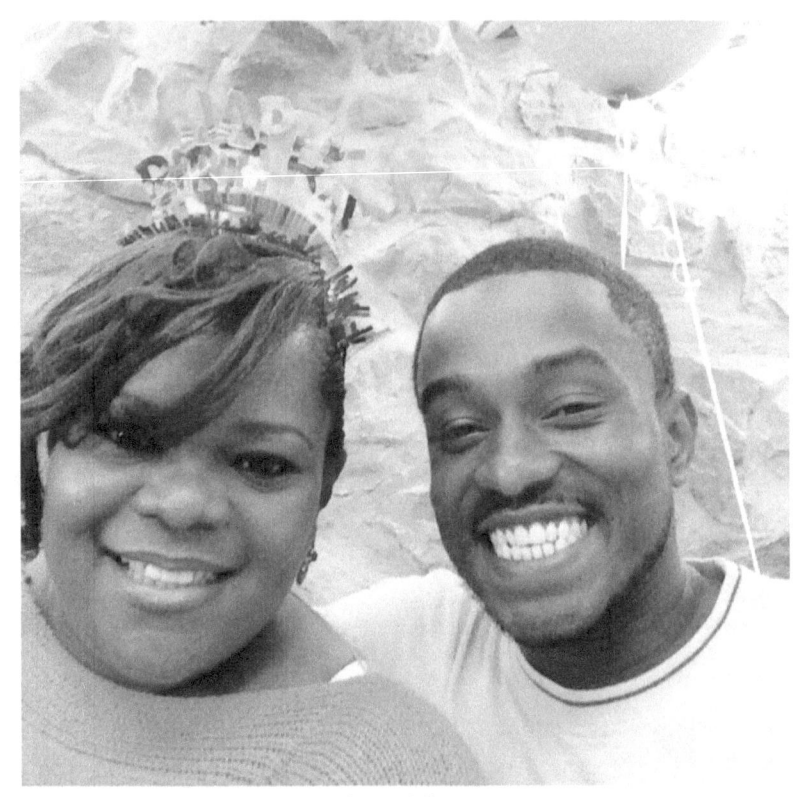

My Son, Xiome

JUMBLED AND CONFUSED

Ok this is just one of those things that we all experience whether you had a brain aneurysm or not. It is thinking one thing and saying something completely different. I often know what I want to say, but my brain won't cooperate and I find myself saying things that make no sense to the listener. While we all may go through this at one point or another, the reality is for an Annie survivor, it can happen daily, hourly and even moment to moment.

Why? That is a good question, the fact is we have had some circuits that were fried for lack of a better phrase. Let's face it, to the medical community we had a stroke. I know that is hard to hear, but that is the designation for an Aneurysm. That was something I did not know until many years later.

When I tried to apply for life insurance shortly after having the Annie, I was turned downed because I was too new out of the hospital! Imagine that, all I wanted was to protect my family should I expire, and no one wanted to help me do that in the insurance industry. I later learned that once I had been 5 years out, I could re-apply and get coverage. Of course, I did just that!

Audrey has no insurance, and lives with the fear that she will not leave anything to her husband or children. She's only 2 years out. I understand her fears. This is that moment when a conversation with everyone from insurance, to medical treatments, and even caretakers requires dialog. A re-evaluation of how you handle Annie survivors and what is considered prudent would be a good start. We deserve specialized care and support for our condition! It is hard enough to live with this fear that it could happen again and that we may not be so lucky next time. But to also add insult to injury by telling us we cannot qualify with our pre-existing condition is tantamount to abuse!

But I digress, the jumbled or confused conversations or actions are a part of daily life. I recall my sister seeing a picture of my granddaughter and she asked me if I remember my son looking the same way as a child? I said yes, and began speaking jumbled words to her. She calmly told me to stop and try to get some rest, because I was not making sense. She put me at ease, because I have learned to let my support systems help me when I cannot help myself. You should do the same thing, because they can recognize when you are not acting or speaking correctly. I can look at an object and try to call its name, only to have something completely wrong come out of my mouth! It is the most frustrating thing you can ever image. Where are my thoughts, why did I say that? I can see people almost stop, frozen with fear that something is wrong, and then they calm down and take control. To the Annie survivor, just go with the flow, to the caregivers, THANK YOU for recognizing the issue, and helping!

SLURRED SPEECH

So jumbled and confused speech is an issue, but it is something much more critical to recognize. It is the drooping of your mouth on one side and struggling to produce words clearly. I know I said this was not a book about what causes Aneurysms, but slurred speech is important and must be discussed.

One of the more significant symptoms of a possible Brain Aneurysm is slurred speech. There are other symptoms but for the sake of this chapter, I want to focus on this one.

Yes, it is always wise to ere on the side of caution and go the hospital if a Brain Aneurysm survivor displays slurred speech. It could be a sign that something is happening that needs medical attention. Even after 10 years, I still have moments of slurred speech. For me they come when I am overly tired. It is my clear sign that I need to stop what I am doing and laydown to rest, NOW! Luckily after years of running straight to the emergency room and undergoing multiple tests, some very painful, I have begun to learn that a good night of rest will do the trick. AGAIN, I state that it has come after 10 years of improving physically and healing emotionally! But know that my support system is so in tune with me that they would not allow me to sleep if they suspected something more serious.

As any Annie survivor has learned, there are these warning signs that you are doing too much. For me the slurred speech that comes without warning, is that sign. Sometimes I don't even realize I am doing it. While I think I am speaking clearly, I am quickly told that my mouth is drooping and the words I release are far from coherent. In my effort to push through I slow down my breathing and begin to utter the words with each breath. That is something I was taught in physical therapy when I was learning how to communicate again. Funny that I remember that at those times. I inhaled deeply then without stopping I exhaled and simultaneously spoke, "I said, I am tired." Finally, the sentence is complete, and all at once I realize my lips are not working properly. It is almost like they have gone to sleep on me! Without being told I get up and turn toward the bedroom. Knowing that it is time to rest, I reluctantly lie down for what I think will be a few moments. My body almost instinctively shuts down and I end up sleeping for a few hours!

Juanita, another survivor says her slurred speech happens when she is at work. On really busy days the stress can cause her speech to slur when she is over doing it. She was lucky that after her rupture she could return to work, but she says it is a daily struggle and she wonders how long she can continue to work.

For those of us who had to endure physical therapy, you will find yourself constantly reverting to the regimen you learned while there. You will find that your speech therapy, which is a part of the physical therapy process will prove invaluable in the long run. Although I must admit I didn't feel this way at the time.

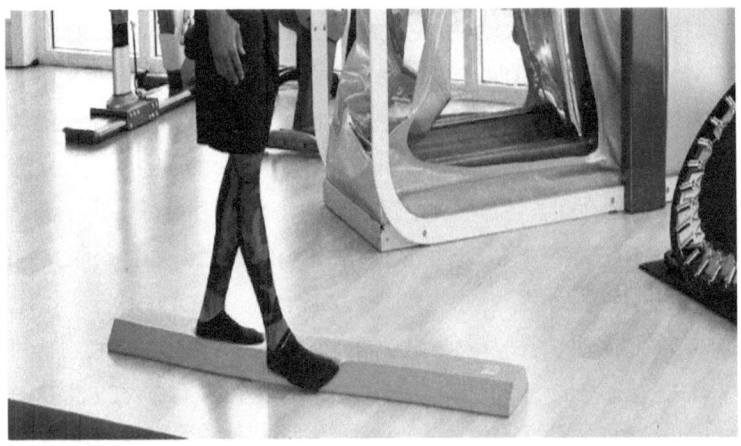

WALKING

Wow, all I can say is "Wow!" I was never a clumsy person, never had difficulty walking in heels or even running. However, one of the great gifts left to me after this Annie, is the inability to walk without tripping over my feet! One of the many things I took for granted was the ability to walk in a very statuesque manner. It was something that came naturally to me, or maybe I just picked it up from my 3 sisters who all walk with authority and confidence. It is a sight to see! Each one has a graceful confidence when they walk into a room! I always envied that skill about them. Nonetheless, when that ability was taken away, I understood how far I had fallen.

Who knew that walking was such a process? I mean all you need to do is put one foot in front of the other, right? Well I can tell you that most of Annie survivors I have met, including myself, all suffer with walking issues. Some of us suffer more than others. If that wasn't enough I find myself thinking about the steps I took as I used to be. A flat foot placed firmly on the ground, heel to toe, heel to toe. Now that I had that down to a science, here is the reality. I cannot walk in heels any longer! For a woman like myself that is a crushing fact of life! I have become quite comfortable in sneakers, flats, and bare feet if that is an option. My ability to walk as my sisters do, you know, much like a diva in command of all that she surveys, was gone. Another reminder of my new reality, that life has changed!

I walk with a slower gate, almost like a shuffle. I can trip over my own two feet sometimes. This was something left over from the Aneurysm. You see I had to learn how to walk and talk again immediately upon my being released from the hospital. Instead of going home and recuperating from there, I had to go straight to rehab. I could not pass go or collect my $200, as they play in the monopoly game. It was overwhelming to accept that I was now in this season of life. When I look back at that time, I am confounded by two facts: The first being that I can remember that time clearly, and the second is that I could not believe how much effort it took to do the simplest things like walking.

At the time I also hated everyone and everything around me. It wasn't fair what was happening, or so I thought. This is where the caregivers/support team came in handy. For me my sister Linda, was a God-send. She simply told me to put one foot in front of the other and keep it moving! At the time, I thought she had no idea what I was going through or how I was feeling, but today I realize she told me just what I needed to hear. She understood that this phase of life was about faith, and trust in God that all would work itself out in time. Her belief helped me to increase my faith in the process. It also helped my determination to stop feeling sorry for myself and 'get it done!' Remember that something so simple to you all can be a major obstacle to the survivor. Be the support that we need and let us lean on you until we are steady again.

This was a season of assurance!

CHAPTER 14

VISION CHANGES

Now let's dive into this realm. You see, vision changes are often dramatic, and hard to deal with. You see, when I had my rupture, I was wearing contact lenses. Funny now that I am writing this, I wonder if the doctors knew that and if they removed my lenses before surgery. You see my rupture was behind my right eye, which meant my vision took a major hit!

I remember the first time I went to the eye doctor, it was somewhat funny how many doctors all want to look into your eyes to see if they can see the coil in position. They literally would ask if they could look into my eyes, not for the exam purposes, but instead to get a first-hand look at a survivor's eye to see the leftovers. I felt like I was a science project and they had to confirm their findings. Sometimes it was no big deal, but then they would shine that light directly into my eye and it felt like someone was stabbing me with a knife. Then it had to stop, immediately. But I digress…back to the chapter at hand.

Vision changes come with the realization that any strong type of light will bother our eyes now. This new sensitivity to light can be painful at times, and almost always blurs the sight directly in front of us. We often wear shades, or squint not to be cool or to give the 'side-eye,' but to stop the pain. The physiological response of fight or flight becomes exponentially stronger with Annie Survivors. With Allen, he has mastered his response, by not going out until the sunsets. Mary wears her sunglasses all the time, she can't even handle a lamp or a television light. I myself, always wear sunglasses outside until sunset, and even the headlights of an oncoming vehicle can cause major pain and has eliminated night time driving.

The doctors never mentioned to us that our vision would be significantly impacted, so I wanted to make sure you that know it could happen. Have your eyes checked every 6 months or so, because changes occur quickly.

Oh and invest in a good pair of sunglasses to protect you from the sunlight.

It must be known and understood that what affects some in minor ways, may well affect the survivor in a more heightened way! A typical cold is not a just cold, but could in fact become a full-blown flu! When we have a headache, it may well be a migraine. So as caregivers be cognizant of the magnitude of our issues. Know that we are not being dramatic although I have been told I have a flare for it, I assure you the issue is real.

I tried to share with you all the things that have affected me or other Annie survivors so you too, can be prepared. Not every survivor has outward indicators of what has happened, like me. But know that we are thoroughly impaired by this event. Whether you're the caregiver or the survivor, there are changes that have occurred and you must find the right way to deal with them.

Had this book been available 10 years ago, I might not have had such a hard time explaining what I was feeling. It wasn't until I began to document my experiences that it started to make sense. I must also admit that my monthly support group was extremely helpful in putting a voice to situations I was going through. Meeting other survivors, sharing our ups and downs, and finding ways to grow into this new life was so cathartic! Perhaps your own story could be of help to someone else. Isn't that what life should be all about, helping others in whatever way you can?

I hope I have opened-up your eyes to what we Annie Survivors go through daily. It is a constant struggle and we do our best to be good at life now. The caregivers are the most important aspect of our survival, and must continue to play an integral role in our lives now.

There is one fact that we survivors must take away from this book, this life, this experience that has overtaken us, and that is this...We are here! In whatever capacity, or strength we have left, we are here! And that is the best encouragement I can offer! When the days get tough, when the pain is unbearable, when people upset you, remember YOU ARE HERE! You are a miracle, a gift from God who gave you a second chance! Now go conquer the world, go find your place, and most of all LIVE!

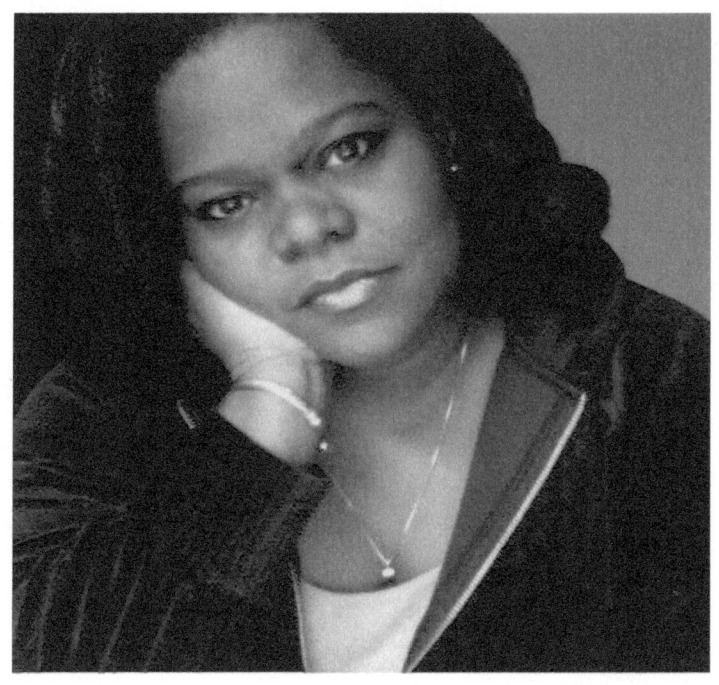

Penny Freeman – Ruptured Brain Aneurysm Survivor!

HELPFUL RESOURCES

- The Brain Aneurysm Foundation – http://www.bafound.org

- Emory Hospital Brain Aneurysm Support Group - Regina Carder (404) 712-5795 - Regina.Carder@emoryhealthcare.org

- John Hopkins Brain Aneurysm Support Group - https://www.hopkinsmedicine.org/neurology_neurosurgery/centers_clinics/aneurysm/support_group.html

- Joe Niekro Foundation - http://www.joeniekrofoundation.com/

- Brain Aneurysm Support Community - http://www.bafsupport.org/

- Emory Hospital Brain Aneurysm Support Group https://www.emoryhealthcare.org/emory-clinic/neurosurgery/support-groups.html

www.ingramcontent.com/pod-product-compliance
Lightning Source LLC
Chambersburg PA
CBHW021451210526
45463CB00002B/729